CODY SMITH

8 Weeks to 200 Consecutive Lunges

Build Stronger Legs by Working Your Glutes, Quads, Lower Back, and Hamstrings | at Home Workouts | No Gym Required |

First edition

ISBN: 978-1-952381-17-1

This book was professionally typeset on Reedsy.
Find out more at reedsy.com

Contents

Before You Begin

Hey reader, thanks for grabbing a copy of the book.

If you are looking to pair this workout program with a complimentary guide to shed weight and boost your growth hormones to build more muscle faster, then I've got you covered.

Seems crazy to do both at the same time, but you can.

Better still, it is stupid easy.

Oh, and it is free. You can do this method anytime you want, anywhere for the rest of your life.

I usually sell this information, but I want you to have it.

You can get a copy from your cell phone from a simple text.

Seriously, get your phone out and text BOOST to (678) 506-7543.

Cheers!

Introduction - How to Use This Book

Lunges are by far my favorite lower body exercise.

They can strengthen and tone your legs and it does not take much before your legs feel like they are on fire.

But as our lifestyle becomes more sedentary, with desk jobs, long commutes to work, and the ability to have just about anything delivered to your front door, keeping your legs in good shape has never been more important.

So whether you're looking to just get a great workout as you shoot for a goal, looking to tone your legs, or need some secret sauce to beat your current lunge PR, this program is for you.

Sadly, you would be hard pressed to find a lot of people even in a gym who can do even 50 consecutive lunges without falling to the ground unable to get up.

But we are not here to shoot for a mere 50. We are going straight for 200 consecutive leg crushers.

We are hitting 3 digits here or we're going home. All or nothing baby.

And that's exactly what you're going to find here in this 8-week program.

Sure, you could do lunges on your own, try and knock out as many as possible every day and work your way to 200 but you are either going to fall short or give up before you even get there.

What you need is strategically designed workouts for your current fitness level that challenge you just enough without killing you. Each workout will push you for the proper progression to make steady gains along the way. This program is structured to take all the guesswork out of your journey to 200 consecutive lunges.

And these workouts that can literally be completed anywhere.

Your journey begins with an initial lunge assessment to find out where your current max is. Afterwards, you will know exactly where to start in the program.

Once you complete the entire program, you will have earned the right to attempt crushing 200 consecutive lunges.

Some people knock it out on their first try. Others will not and will need to hack it a few more weeks before trying again.

Now, I will warn you, these workouts can feel very repetitive at times. Far too often people look for variety and complexity to see results when really the simplest of approaches is best.
   100 lunges variations and off the wall workout routines are not what is going to get you to the results you want. Showing up and putting in the work; that is where the real bacon is.

Some of you will not need the entire 8 weeks. Others will need more than 8 weeks. Either way is perfectly fine and doesn't mean the program doesn't work, it just means everyone comes from a different level of fitness.

8 weeks is not some magical number that will work for every single person. 8 weeks is the average amount of time it will take the average person to reach 200 consecutive lunges so do not get too caught up in the timeline. It will take you however long that it takes you.

What I can promise you is if you put in the work, you will see the results.

Up next is the initial assessment. Get after it, champ.

Initial Lunge Assessment

This is the first step into your incredible journey to doing 200 consecutive lunges. It will be hard but manageable as you embark on something that very few people on the face of the earth have ever accomplished.

We are going to start out with a lunge assessment to determine where you should start in the program.

Make sure you are doing full lunges going all the way through the motion. Proper form is key to getting the most out of this exercise so I'll quickly go over how to properly perform a lunge with stationary lunges or walking lunges.

For stationary lunges:

You are going to start the exercise by standing with your feet hip-width apart. Begin the lunge by taking a step forward starting with your right leg striking the ground with your heel first. Lower your body until the right thigh is parallel to the ground. You will know you've reached the full descend if your left knee lightly taps the ground. Press with the right foot to drive back to the start position. Repeat for the left leg. That is one rep.

For walking lunges:

You are going to start the exercise by standing with your feet hip-width apart.

Begin the lunge by taking a step forward starting with your right leg striking the ground with your heel first. Lower your body until the right thigh is parallel to the ground. You will know you've reached the full descend if your left knee lightly taps the ground. At the lowest point of the lunge, instead of returning to the start position, press with your right foot as you shift your weight forward. Rise up as you bring your left or back foot forward to initiate the next lunge stepping forward with the opposite foot. That is one rep.

Throughout the motion, your back should not bend.

Go ahead and get into the starting position if you have not done so already. Make sure you have room to do either stationary or walking lunges, whichever you choose.

You are going to complete as many correct lunges as you can without stopping.

Once you are done, write down the number of fully completed lunges below and head to the post assessment results section.

Note: If this is the first assessment, you will write your assessment number in the '1st assessment' row. When you come back to do another assessment, you write in your completed number of reps in the respective row depending on how many assessments you have completed.

_____ reps: 1st assessment

_____ reps: 2nd assessment

_____ reps: 3rd assessment

_____ reps: 4th assessment

_____ reps: 5th assessment

_____ reps: 6th assessment

_____ reps: 7th assessment

_____ reps: 8th assessment

_____ reps: 9th assessment

_____ reps: 10th assessment

_____ reps: 11th assessment

_____ reps: 12th assessment

_____ reps: 13th assessment

_____ reps: 14th assessment

_____ reps: 15th assessment

_____ reps: 16th assessment

_____ reps: 17th assessment

_____ reps: 18th assessment

_____ reps: 19th assessment

_____ reps: 20th assessment

Post-Assessment Results

So... how did you do?

Were you surprised with how many you did or were you underwhelmed and disappointed that you did not do so hot?

Do not beat yourself up. This is simply a baseline for you to start from.

Go ahead and jog your memory of your assessment score.

With that score in mind, you are now going to be directed to your workout grouping based on your score.

Do not get too caught up in the name of each group of workouts, these are just fun names to identify which group you are currently in. If you do not like your current group name, do not worry, stick with the program long enough and you will be out of that group in no time and into another group whose name you probably will not like either.

Before I go into informing you of your baseline workout, I recommend leaving a day between now and hitting your first workout to recover from your assessment. However, you do not have to if you are feeling gung-ho and want to go ahead and knock out your first workout.

- If you did 10, you will start in the Novice Group.
- If you did between 11 and 20, you will start in the Newb Group.
- If you did between 21 and 30, you will start in the Greenhorn Group.
- If you did between 31 and 40, you will start in the Cub Group.
- If you did between 41 and 50, you will start in the Rookie Group.
- If you did between 51 and 60, you will start in the Pleb Group.
- If you did between 61 and 70, you will start in the Gorilla Group.
- If you did between 71 and 80, you will start in the Viking Group.
- If you did between 81 and 90, you will start in the Elite Group.
- If you did between 91 and 100, you will start in the Commando Group.
- If you did between 101 and 110, you will start in the Veteran Group.
- If you did greater than 110, you will start in the Nuclear Group.

Now that you know your group, you know where you will begin for your next workout.

In your group, you will start with workout 1 followed by workout 2 and 3.

For example, let's say you completed 23 reps and you were going to workout Monday, Wednesday and Friday. That would put you in the Greenhorn Group with workout 1 on Monday, Workout 2 on Wednesday, and workout 3 on Friday.

The following week, you would start with greenhorn Group Workout 4 followed by 5 and 6.

Simple enough.

Great job on your assessment and get ready for your first workout.

Workout Completion Checklist

Check off your workouts as you complete them:

_____Novice Group Workout 1

_____Novice Group Workout 2

_____Novice Group Workout 3

_____Novice Group Workout 4

_____Novice Group Workout 5

_____Novice Group Workout 6

_____Newb Group Workout 1

_____Newb Group Workout 2

_____Newb Group Workout 3

_____Newb Group Workout 4

_____Newb Group Workout 5

_____Newb Group Workout 6

_____Greenhorn Group Workout 1

_____Greenhorn Group Workout 2

_____Greenhorn Group Workout 3

_____Greenhorn Group Workout 4

_____Greenhorn Group Workout 5

_____Greenhorn Group Workout 6

_____Cub Group Workout 1

_____Cub Group Workout 2

_____Cub Group Workout 3

_____Cub Group Workout 4

_____Cub Group Workout 5

_____Cub Group Workout 6

_____Rookie Group Workout 1

_____Rookie Group Workout 2

_____Rookie Group Workout 3

_____Rookie Group Workout 4

_____Rookie Group Workout 5

_____Rookie Group Workout 6

_____Pleb Group Workout 1

_____Pleb Group Workout 2

_____Pleb Group Workout 3

_____Pleb Group Workout 4

_____Pleb Group Workout 5

_____Pleb Group Workout 6

_____Gorilla Group Workout 1

_____Gorilla Group Workout 2

_____Gorilla Group Workout 3

_____Gorilla Group Workout 4

_____Gorilla Group Workout 5

_____Gorilla Group Workout 6

_____Viking Group Workout 1

_____Viking Group Workout 2

_____Viking Group Workout 3

_____Viking Group Workout 4

_____Viking Group Workout 5

_____Viking Group Workout 6

_____Elite Group Workout 1

_____Elite Group Workout 2

_____Elite Group Workout 3

_____Elite Group Workout 4

_____Elite Group Workout 5

_____Elite Group Workout 6

_____Commando Group Workout 1

_____Commando Group Workout 2

_____Commando Group Workout 3

_____Commando Group Workout 4

_____Commando Group Workout 5

_____Commando Group Workout 6

_____Veteran Group Workout 1

_____Veteran Group Workout 2

_____Veteran Group Workout 3

_____Veteran Group Workout 4

_____Veteran Group Workout 5

_____Veteran Group Workout 6

_____Nuclear Group Workout 1

_____Nuclear Group Workout 2

_____Nuclear Group Workout 3

_____Nuclear Group Workout 4

_____Nuclear Group Workout 5

_____Nuclear Group Workout 6

_____Attempting 200 Consecutive Lunges

_____Completed 200 Consecutive Lunges: _____ reps.

Pre & Post Program Measurements

The following measurements are 100% optional and are not required to start or finish the program. I know some people will be curious to know other areas that are positively affected by achieving 200 consecutive lunges.

Starting weight: _____

Starting lunge rep max: _____

Starting lunge max: _____

Starting deadlift max: _____

Starting leg press max: _____

Starting right thigh measurement: _____

Ending weight: _____

Ending lunge rep max: _____

Ending lunge max: _____

Ending deadlift max: _____

Ending leg press max: _____

Ending right thigh measurement: _____

Novice Group Workouts

Novice Group Workout 1

Welcome to the Novice Group Workout 1.

For this workout, you have 6 sets with 60 seconds of rest between each set.

Remember to focus on proper form throughout your sets.

Sets:

1. 5 lunges
2. 5 lunges
3. 5 lunges
4. 5 lunges
5. 5 lunges
6. Max out: perform as many lunges as you can.

Max reps: _____

If you completed this workout, head to Novice Group Workout 2 for your next session. If not, stick with this one until you complete it.

Glasses of water drank today: 1-2-3-4-5-6-7-8-9-10

Hours of sleep last night: 1-2-3-4-5-6-7-8-9-10

Diet: junk food—————semi-healthy—————healthy

Novice Group Workout 2

Welcome to the Novice Group Workout 2.

For this workout, you have 6 sets with 60 seconds of rest between each set.

Remember to focus on proper form throughout your sets.

Sets:

1. 7 lunges
2. 7 lunges
3. 7 lunges
4. 7 lunges
5. 7 lunges
6. Max out: perform as many lunges as you can.

Max reps: _____

If you completed this workout, head to Novice Group Workout 3 for your next session. If not, stick with this one until you complete it.

Glasses of water drank today: 1-2-3-4-5-6-7-8-9-10

Hours of sleep last night: 1-2-3-4-5-6-7-8-9-10

Diet: junk food—————semi-healthy—————healthy

Novice Group Workout 3

Welcome to the Novice Group Workout 3.

For this workout, you have 6 sets with 90 seconds of rest between each set.

Remember to focus on proper form throughout your sets.

Sets:

1. 8 lunges
2. 8 lunges
3. 8 lunges
4. 8 lunges
5. 8 lunges
6. Max out: perform as many lunges as you can.

Max reps: _____

If you completed this workout, head to Novice Group Workout 4 for your next session. If not, stick with this one until you complete it.

Glasses of water drank today: 1-2-3-4-5-6-7-8-9-10

Hours of sleep last night: 1-2-3-4-5-6-7-8-9-10

Diet: junk food—————semi-healthy—————healthy

Novice Group Workout 4

Welcome to the Novice Group Workout 4.

For this workout, you have 6 sets with 60 seconds of rest between each set.

Remember to focus on proper form throughout your sets.

Sets:

1. 10 lunges
2. 10 lunges
3. 10 lunges
4. 10 lunges
5. 10 lunges
6. Max out: perform as many lunges as you can.

Max reps: _____

If you completed this workout, head to Novice Group Workout 5 for your next session. If not, stick with this one until you complete it.

Glasses of water drank today: 1-2-3-4-5-6-7-8-9-10

Hours of sleep last night: 1-2-3-4-5-6-7-8-9-10

Diet: junk food—————semi-healthy—————healthy

Novice Group Workout 5

Welcome to the Novice Group Workout 5.

For this workout, you have 6 sets with 60 seconds of rest between each set.

Remember to focus on proper form throughout your sets.

Sets:

1. 11 lunges
2. 11 lunges
3. 11 lunges
4. 11 lunges
5. 11 lunges
6. Max out: perform as many lunges as you can.

Max reps: _____

If you completed this workout, head to Novice Group Workout 6 for your next session. If not, stick with this one until you complete it.

Glasses of water drank today: 1-2-3-4-5-6-7-8-9-10

Hours of sleep last night: 1-2-3-4-5-6-7-8-9-10

Diet: junk food—————semi-healthy—————healthy

Novice Group Workout 6

Welcome to the Novice Group Workout 6.

For this workout, you have 6 sets with 90 seconds of rest between each set.

Remember to focus on proper form throughout your sets.

Sets:

1. 14 lunges
2. 14 lunges
3. 14 lunges
4. 14 lunges
5. 14 lunges
6. Max out: perform as many lunges as you can.

Max reps: _____

Since this is the end of a two-week period, it is time to redo your lunge assessment to check your progress if you fully completed this workout.

Rest a day and give the assessment a go to see which Group you will be in next.

Glasses of water drank today: 1-2-3-4-5-6-7-8-9-10

Hours of sleep last night: 1-2-3-4-5-6-7-8-9-10

Diet: junk food————semi-healthy————healthy

Newb Group Workouts

Newb Group Workout 1

Welcome to the Newb Group Workout 1.

For this workout, you have 6 sets with 60 seconds of rest between each set.

Remember to focus on proper form throughout your sets.

Sets:

1. 11 lunges
2. 11 lunges
3. 11 lunges
4. 11 lunges
5. 11 lunges
6. Max out: perform as many lunges as you can.

Max reps: _____

If you completed this workout, head to Newb Group Workout 2 for your next session. If not, stick with this one until you complete it.

Glasses of water drank today: 1-2-3-4-5-6-7-8-9-10

Hours of sleep last night: 1-2-3-4-5-6-7-8-9-10

Diet: junk food—————semi-healthy—————healthy

Newb Group Workout 2

Welcome to the Newb Group Workout 2.

For this workout, you have 6 sets with 60 seconds of rest between each set.

Remember to focus on proper form throughout your sets.

Sets:

1. 14 lunges
2. 14 lunges
3. 14 lunges
4. 14 lunges
5. 14 lunges
6. Max out: perform as many lunges as you can.

Max reps: _____

If you completed this workout, head to Newb Group Workout 3 for your next session. If not, stick with this one until you complete it.

Glasses of water drank today: 1-2-3-4-5-6-7-8-9-10

Hours of sleep last night: 1-2-3-4-5-6-7-8-9-10

Diet: junk food————semi-healthy————healthy

Newb Group Workout 3

Welcome to the Newb Group Workout 3.

For this workout, you have 6 sets with 90 seconds of rest between each set.

Remember to focus on proper form throughout your sets.

Sets:

1. 17 lunges
2. 17 lunges
3. 17 lunges
4. 17 lunges
5. 17 lunges
6. Max out: perform as many lunges as you can.

Max reps: _____

If you completed this workout, head to Newb Group Workout 4 for your next session. If not, stick with this one until you complete it.

Glasses of water drank today: 1-2-3-4-5-6-7-8-9-10

Hours of sleep last night: 1-2-3-4-5-6-7-8-9-10

Diet: junk food—————semi-healthy—————healthy

Newb Group Workout 4

Welcome to the Newb Group Workout 4.

For this workout, you have 6 sets with 60 seconds of rest between each set.

Remember to focus on proper form throughout your sets.

Sets:

1. 19 lunges
2. 19 lunges
3. 19 lunges
4. 19 lunges
5. 19 lunges
6. Max out: perform as many lunges as you can.

Max reps: _____

If you completed this workout, head to Newb Group Workout 5 for your next session. If not, stick with this one until you complete it.

Glasses of water drank today: 1-2-3-4-5-6-7-8-9-10

Hours of sleep last night: 1-2-3-4-5-6-7-8-9-10

Diet: junk food—————semi-healthy—————healthy

Newb Group Workout 5

Welcome to the Newb Group Workout 5.

For this workout, you have 6 sets with 60 seconds of rest between each set.

Remember to focus on proper form throughout your sets.

Sets:

1. 21 lunges
2. 21 lunges
3. 21 lunges
4. 21 lunges
5. 21 lunges
6. Max out: perform as many lunges as you can.

Max reps: _____

If you completed this workout, head to Newb Group Workout 6 for your next session. If not, stick with this one until you complete it.

Glasses of water drank today: 1-2-3-4-5-6-7-8-9-10

Hours of sleep last night: 1-2-3-4-5-6-7-8-9-10

Diet: junk food————semi-healthy————healthy

Newb Group Workout 6

Welcome to the Newb Group Workout 6.

For this workout, you have 6 sets with 90 seconds of rest between each set.

Remember to focus on proper form throughout your sets.

Sets:

1. 23 lunges
2. 23 lunges
3. 23 lunges
4. 23 lunges
5. 23 lunges
6. Max out: perform as many lunges as you can.

Max reps: _____

Since this is the end of a two-week period, it is time to redo your lunge assessment to check your progress if you fully completed this workout.

Rest a day and give the assessment a go to see which Group you will be in next.

Glasses of water drank today: 1-2-3-4-5-6-7-8-9-10

Hours of sleep last night: 1-2-3-4-5-6-7-8-9-10

Diet: junk food—————semi-healthy—————healthy

Greenhorn Group Workouts

Greenhorn Group Workout 1

Welcome to the Greenhorn Group Workout 1.

For this workout, you have 6 sets with 60 seconds of rest between each set.

Remember to focus on proper form throughout your sets.

Sets:

1. 19 lunges
2. 19 lunges
3. 19 lunges
4. 19 lunges
5. 19 lunges
6. Max out: perform as many lunges as you can.

Max reps: _____

If you completed this workout, head to Greenhorn Group Workout 2 for your next session. If not, stick with this one until you complete it.

Glasses of water drank today: 1-2-3-4-5-6-7-8-9-10

Hours of sleep last night: 1-2-3-4-5-6-7-8-9-10

Diet: junk food—————semi-healthy—————healthy

Greenhorn Group Workout 2

Welcome to the Greenhorn Group Workout 2.

For this workout, you have 6 sets with 60 seconds of rest between each set.

Remember to focus on proper form throughout your sets.

Sets:

1. 20 lunges
2. 20 lunges
3. 20 lunges
4. 20 lunges
5. 20 lunges
6. Max out: perform as many lunges as you can.

Max reps: _____

If you completed this workout, head to Greenhorn Group Workout 3 for your next session. If not, stick with this one until you complete it.

Glasses of water drank today: 1-2-3-4-5-6-7-8-9-10

Hours of sleep last night: 1-2-3-4-5-6-7-8-9-10

Diet: junk food—————semi-healthy—————healthy

Greenhorn Group Workout 3

Welcome to the Greenhorn Group Workout 3.

For this workout, you have 6 sets with 90 seconds of rest between each set.

Remember to focus on proper form throughout your sets.

Sets:

1. 23 lunges
2. 23 lunges
3. 23 lunges
4. 23 lunges
5. 23 lunges
6. Max out: perform as many lunges as you can.

Max reps: _____

If you completed this workout, head to Greenhorn Group Workout 4 for your next session. If not, stick with this one until you complete it.

Glasses of water drank today: 1-2-3-4-5-6-7-8-9-10

Hours of sleep last night: 1-2-3-4-5-6-7-8-9-10

Diet: junk food————semi-healthy————healthy

Greenhorn Group Workout 4

Welcome to the Greenhorn Group Workout 4.

For this workout, you have 6 sets with 60 seconds of rest between each set.

Remember to focus on proper form throughout your sets.

Sets:

1. 25 lunges
2. 25 lunges
3. 25 lunges
4. 25 lunges
5. 25 lunges
6. Max out: perform as many lunges as you can.

Max reps: _____

If you completed this workout, head to Greenhorn Group Workout 5 for your next session. If not, stick with this one until you complete it.

Glasses of water drank today: 1-2-3-4-5-6-7-8-9-10

Hours of sleep last night: 1-2-3-4-5-6-7-8-9-10

Diet: junk food—————semi-healthy—————healthy

Greenhorn Group Workout 5

Welcome to the Greenhorn Group Workout 5.

For this workout, you have 6 sets with 60 seconds of rest between each set.

Remember to focus on proper form throughout your sets.

Sets:

1. 28 lunges
2. 28 lunges
3. 28 lunges
4. 28 lunges
5. 28 lunges
6. Max out: perform as many lunges as you can.

Max reps: _____

If you completed this workout, head to Greenhorn Group Workout 6 for your next session. If not, stick with this one until you complete it.

Glasses of water drank today: 1-2-3-4-5-6-7-8-9-10

Hours of sleep last night: 1-2-3-4-5-6-7-8-9-10

Diet: junk food—————semi-healthy—————healthy

Greenhorn Group Workout 6

Welcome to the Greenhorn Group Workout 6.

For this workout, you have 6 sets with 90 seconds of rest between each set.

Remember to focus on proper form throughout your sets.

Sets:

1. 31 lunges
2. 31 lunges
3. 31 lunges
4. 31 lunges
5. 31 lunges
6. Max out: perform as many lunges as you can.

Max reps: _____

Since this is the end of a two-week period, it is time to redo your lunge assessment to check your progress if you fully completed this workout.

Rest a day and give the assessment a go to see which Group you will be in next.

Glasses of water drank today: 1-2-3-4-5-6-7-8-9-10

Hours of sleep last night: 1-2-3-4-5-6-7-8-9-10

Diet: junk food————semi-healthy————healthy

Cub Group Workouts

Cub Group Workout 1

Welcome to the Cub Group Workout 1.

For this workout, you have 6 sets with 60 seconds of rest between each set.

Remember to focus on proper form throughout your sets.

Sets:

1. 23 lunges
2. 23 lunges
3. 23 lunges
4. 23 lunges
5. 23 lunges
6. Max out: perform as many lunges as you can.

Max reps: _____

If you completed this workout, head to Cub Group Workout 2 for your next session. If not, stick with this one until you complete it.

Glasses of water drank today: 1-2-3-4-5-6-7-8-9-10

Hours of sleep last night: 1-2-3-4-5-6-7-8-9-10

Diet: junk food—————semi-healthy—————healthy

Cub Group Workout 2

Welcome to the Cub Group Workout 2.

For this workout, you have 6 sets with 60 seconds of rest between each set.

Remember to focus on proper form throughout your sets.

Sets:

1. 25 lunges
2. 25 lunges
3. 25 lunges
4. 25 lunges
5. 25 lunges
6. Max out: perform as many lunges as you can.

Max reps: _____

If you completed this workout, head to Cub Group Workout 3 for your next session. If not, stick with this one until you complete it.

Glasses of water drank today: 1-2-3-4-5-6-7-8-9-10

Hours of sleep last night: 1-2-3-4-5-6-7-8-9-10

Diet: junk food—————semi-healthy—————healthy

Cub Group Workout 3

Welcome to the Cub Group Workout 3.

For this workout, you have 6 sets with 90 seconds of rest between each set.

Remember to focus on proper form throughout your sets.

Sets:

1. 28 lunges
2. 28 lunges
3. 28 lunges
4. 28 lunges
5. 28 lunges
6. Max out: perform as many lunges as you can.

Max reps: _____

If you completed this workout, head to Cub Group Workout 4 for your next session. If not, stick with this one until you complete it.

Glasses of water drank today: 1-2-3-4-5-6-7-8-9-10

Hours of sleep last night: 1-2-3-4-5-6-7-8-9-10

Diet: junk food————semi-healthy————healthy

Cub Group Workout 4

Welcome to the Cub Group Workout 4.

For this workout, you have 6 sets with 60 seconds of rest between each set.

Remember to focus on proper form throughout your sets.

Sets:

1. 31 lunges
2. 31 lunges
3. 31 lunges
4. 31 lunges
5. 31 lunges
6. Max out: perform as many lunges as you can.

Max reps: _____

If you completed this workout, head to Cub Group Workout 5 for your next session. If not, stick with this one until you complete it.

Glasses of water drank today: 1-2-3-4-5-6-7-8-9-10

Hours of sleep last night: 1-2-3-4-5-6-7-8-9-10

Diet: junk food————semi-healthy————healthy

Cub Group Workout 5

Welcome to the Cub Group Workout 5.

For this workout, you have 6 sets with 60 seconds of rest between each set.

Remember to focus on proper form throughout your sets.

Sets:

1. 34 lunges
2. 34 lunges
3. 34 lunges
4. 34 lunges
5. 34 lunges
6. Max out: perform as many lunges as you can.

Max reps: _____

If you completed this workout, head to Cub Group Workout 6 for your next session. If not, stick with this one until you complete it.

Glasses of water drank today: 1-2-3-4-5-6-7-8-9-10

Hours of sleep last night: 1-2-3-4-5-6-7-8-9-10

Diet: junk food————semi-healthy————healthy

Cub Group Workout 6

Welcome to the Cub Group Workout 6.

For this workout, you have 6 sets with 90 seconds of rest between each set.

Remember to focus on proper form throughout your sets.

Sets:

1. 37 lunges
2. 37 lunges
3. 37 lunges
4. 37 lunges
5. 37 lunges
6. Max out: perform as many lunges as you can.

Max reps: _____

Since this is the end of a two-week period, it is time to redo your lunge assessment to check your progress if you fully completed this workout.

Rest a day and give the assessment a go to see which Group you will be in next.

Glasses of water drank today: 1-2-3-4-5-6-7-8-9-10

Hours of sleep last night: 1-2-3-4-5-6-7-8-9-10

Diet: junk food————semi-healthy————healthy

Rookie Group Workouts

Rookie Group Workout 1

Welcome to the Rookie Group Workout 1.

For this workout, you have 6 sets with 60 seconds of rest between each set.

Remember to focus on proper form throughout your sets.

Sets:

1. 28 lunges
2. 28 lunges
3. 28 lunges
4. 28 lunges
5. 28 lunges
6. Max out: perform as many lunges as you can.

Max reps: _____

If you completed this workout, head to Cub Group Workout 2 for your next session. If not, stick with this one until you complete it.

Glasses of water drank today: 1-2-3-4-5-6-7-8-9-10

Hours of sleep last night: 1-2-3-4-5-6-7-8-9-10

Diet: junk food————semi-healthy————healthy

Rookie Group Workout 2

Welcome to the Rookie Group Workout 2.

For this workout, you have 6 sets with 60 seconds of rest between each set.

Remember to focus on proper form throughout your sets.

Sets:

1. 31 lunges
2. 31 lunges
3. 31 lunges
4. 31 lunges
5. 31 lunges
6. Max out: perform as many lunges as you can.

Max reps: _____

If you completed this workout, head to Rookie Group Workout 3 for your next session. If not, stick with this one until you complete it.

Glasses of water drank today: 1-2-3-4-5-6-7-8-9-10

Hours of sleep last night: 1-2-3-4-5-6-7-8-9-10

Diet: junk food————semi-healthy————healthy

Rookie Group Workout 3

Welcome to the Rookie Group Workout 3.

For this workout, you have 6 sets with 90 seconds of rest between each set.

Remember to focus on proper form throughout your sets.

Sets:

1. 34 lunges
2. 34 lunges
3. 34 lunges
4. 34 lunges
5. 34 lunges
6. Max out: perform as many lunges as you can.

Max reps: _____

If you completed this workout, head to Rookie Group Workout 4 for your next session. If not, stick with this one until you complete it.

Glasses of water drank today: 1-2-3-4-5-6-7-8-9-10

Hours of sleep last night: 1-2-3-4-5-6-7-8-9-10

Diet: junk food—————semi-healthy—————healthy

Rookie Group Workout 4

Welcome to the Rookie Group Workout 4.

For this workout, you have 6 sets with 60 seconds of rest between each set.

Remember to focus on proper form throughout your sets.

Sets:

1. 37 lunges
2. 37 lunges
3. 37 lunges
4. 37 lunges
5. 37 lunges
6. Max out: perform as many lunges as you can.

Max reps: _____

If you completed this workout, head to Rookie Group Workout 5 for your next session. If not, stick with this one until you complete it.

Glasses of water drank today: 1-2-3-4-5-6-7-8-9-10

Hours of sleep last night: 1-2-3-4-5-6-7-8-9-10

Diet: junk food—————semi-healthy—————healthy

Rookie Group Workout 5

Welcome to the Rookie Group Workout 5.

For this workout, you have 6 sets with 60 seconds of rest between each set.

Remember to focus on proper form throughout your sets.

Sets:

1. 43 lunges
2. 43 lunges
3. 43 lunges
4. 43 lunges
5. 43 lunges
6. Max out: perform as many lunges as you can.

Max reps: _____

If you completed this workout, head to Rookie Group Workout 6 for your next session. If not, stick with this one until you complete it.

Glasses of water drank today: 1-2-3-4-5-6-7-8-9-10

Hours of sleep last night: 1-2-3-4-5-6-7-8-9-10

Diet: junk food———————semi-healthy———————healthy

Rookie Group Workout 6

Welcome to the Rookie Group Workout 6.

For this workout, you have 6 sets with 90 seconds of rest between each set.

Remember to focus on proper form throughout your sets.

Sets:

1. 49 lunges
2. 49 lunges
3. 49 lunges
4. 49 lunges
5. 49 lunges
6. Max out: perform as many lunges as you can.

Max reps: _____

Since this is the end of a two-week period, it is time to redo your lunge assessment to check your progress if you fully completed this workout.

Rest a day and give the assessment a go to see which Group you will be in next.

Glasses of water drank today: 1-2-3-4-5-6-7-8-9-10

Hours of sleep last night: 1-2-3-4-5-6-7-8-9-10

Diet: junk food—————semi-healthy—————healthy

Pleb Group Workouts

Pleb Group Workout 1

Welcome to the Pleb Group Workout 1.

For this workout, you have 6 sets with 60 seconds of rest between each set.

Remember to focus on proper form throughout your sets.

Sets:

1. 34 lunges
2. 34 lunges
3. 34 lunges
4. 34 lunges
5. 34 lunges
6. Max out: perform as many lunges as you can.

Max reps: _____

If you completed this workout, head to Pleb Group Workout 2 for your next session. If not, stick with this one until you complete it.

Glasses of water drank today: 1-2-3-4-5-6-7-8-9-10

Hours of sleep last night: 1-2-3-4-5-6-7-8-9-10

Diet: junk food—————semi-healthy—————healthy

Pleb Group Workout 2

Welcome to the Pleb Group Workout 2.

For this workout, you have 6 sets with 60 seconds of rest between each set.

Remember to focus on proper form throughout your sets.

Sets:

1. 38 lunges
2. 38 lunges
3. 38 lunges
4. 38 lunges
5. 38 lunges
6. Max out: perform as many lunges as you can.

Max reps: _____

If you completed this workout, head to Pleb Group Workout 3 for your next session. If not, stick with this one until you complete it.

Glasses of water drank today: 1-2-3-4-5-6-7-8-9-10

Hours of sleep last night: 1-2-3-4-5-6-7-8-9-10

Diet: junk food————semi-healthy————healthy

Pleb Group Workout 3

Welcome to the Pleb Group Workout 3.

For this workout, you have 6 sets with 90 seconds of rest between each set.

Remember to focus on proper form throughout your sets.

Sets:

1. 42 lunges
2. 42 lunges
3. 42 lunges
4. 42 lunges
5. 42 lunges
6. Max out: perform as many lunges as you can.

Max reps: _____

If you completed this workout, head to Pleb Group Workout 4 for your next session. If not, stick with this one until you complete it.

Glasses of water drank today: 1-2-3-4-5-6-7-8-9-10

Hours of sleep last night: 1-2-3-4-5-6-7-8-9-10

Diet: junk food————semi-healthy————healthy

Pleb Group Workout 4

Welcome to the Pleb Group Workout 4.

For this workout, you have 6 sets with 60 seconds of rest between each set.

Remember to focus on proper form throughout your sets.

Sets:

1. 45 lunges
2. 45 lunges
3. 45 lunges
4. 45 lunges
5. 45 lunges
6. Max out: perform as many lunges as you can.

Max reps: _____

If you completed this workout, head to Pleb Group Workout 5 for your next session. If not, stick with this one until you complete it.

Glasses of water drank today: 1-2-3-4-5-6-7-8-9-10

Hours of sleep last night: 1-2-3-4-5-6-7-8-9-10

Diet: junk food—————semi-healthy—————healthy

Pleb Group Workout 5

Welcome to the Pleb Group Workout 5.

For this workout, you have 6 sets with 60 seconds of rest between each set.

Remember to focus on proper form throughout your sets.

Sets:

1. 53 lunges
2. 53 lunges
3. 53 lunges
4. 53 lunges
5. 53 lunges
6. Max out: perform as many lunges as you can.

Max reps: _____

If you completed this workout, head to Pleb Group Workout 6 for your next session. If not, stick with this one until you complete it.

Glasses of water drank today: 1-2-3-4-5-6-7-8-9-10

Hours of sleep last night: 1-2-3-4-5-6-7-8-9-10

Diet: junk food—————semi-healthy—————healthy

Pleb Group Workout 6

Welcome to the Pleb Group Workout 6.

For this workout, you have 6 sets with 90 seconds of rest between each set.

Remember to focus on proper form throughout your sets.

Sets:

1. 61 lunges
2. 61 lunges
3. 61 lunges
4. 61 lunges
5. 61 lunges
6. Max out: perform as many lunges as you can.

Max reps: _____

Since this is the end of a two-week period, it is time to redo your lunge assessment to check your progress if you fully completed this workout.

Rest a day and give the assessment a go to see which Group you will be in next.

Glasses of water drank today: 1-2-3-4-5-6-7-8-9-10

Hours of sleep last night: 1-2-3-4-5-6-7-8-9-10

Diet: junk food————semi-healthy————healthy

Gorilla Group Workouts

Gorilla Group Workout 1

Welcome to the Gorilla Group Workout 1.

For this workout, you have 6 sets with 120 seconds of rest between each set.

Remember to focus on proper form throughout your sets.

Sets:

1. 42 lunges
2. 42 lunges
3. 42 lunges
4. 42 lunges
5. 42 lunges
6. Max out: perform as many lunges as you can.

Max reps: _____

If you completed this workout, head to Gorilla Group Workout 2 for your next session. If not, stick with this one until you complete it.

Glasses of water drank today: 1-2-3-4-5-6-7-8-9-10

Hours of sleep last night: 1-2-3-4-5-6-7-8-9-10

Diet: junk food—————semi-healthy—————healthy

Gorilla Group Workout 2

Welcome to the Gorilla Group Workout 2.

For this workout, you have 9 sets with 90 seconds of rest between each set.

Remember to focus on proper form throughout your sets.

Sets:

1. 28 lunges
2. 28 lunges
3. 28 lunges
4. 28 lunges
5. 28 lunges
6. 28 lunges
7. 28 lunges
8. 28 lunges
9. Max out: perform as many lunges as you can.

Max reps: _____

If you completed this workout, head to Gorilla Group Workout 3 for your next session. If not, stick with this one until you complete it.

Glasses of water drank today: 1-2-3-4-5-6-7-8-9-10

Hours of sleep last night: 1-2-3-4-5-6-7-8-9-10

Diet: junk food————semi-healthy————healthy

Gorilla Group Workout 3

Welcome to the Gorilla Group Workout 3.

For this workout, you have 9 sets with 90 seconds of rest between each set.

Remember to focus on proper form throughout your sets.

Sets:

1. 30 lunges
2. 30 lunges
3. 30 lunges
4. 30 lunges
5. 30 lunges
6. 30 lunges
7. 30 lunges
8. 30 lunges
9. Max out: perform as many lunges as you can.

Max reps: _____

If you completed this workout, head to Gorilla Group Workout 4 for your next session. If not, stick with this one until you complete it.

Glasses of water drank today: 1-2-3-4-5-6-7-8-9-10

Hours of sleep last night: 1-2-3-4-5-6-7-8-9-10

Diet: junk food————semi-healthy————healthy

Gorilla Group Workout 4

Welcome to the Gorilla Group Workout 4.

For this workout, you have 6 sets with 120 seconds of rest between each set.

Remember to focus on proper form throughout your sets.

Sets:

1. 61 lunges
2. 61 lunges
3. 61 lunges
4. 61 lunges
5. 61 lunges
6. Max out: perform as many lunges as you can.

Max reps: _____

If you completed this workout, head to Gorilla Group Workout 5 for your next session. If not, stick with this one until you complete it.

Glasses of water drank today: 1-2-3-4-5-6-7-8-9-10

Hours of sleep last night: 1-2-3-4-5-6-7-8-9-10

Diet: junk food—————semi-healthy—————healthy

Gorilla Group Workout 5

Welcome to the Gorilla Group Workout 5.

For this workout, you have 10 sets with 90 seconds of rest between each set.

Remember to focus on proper form throughout your sets.

Sets:

1. 35 lunges
2. 35 lunges
3. 35 lunges
4. 35 lunges
5. 35 lunges
6. 35 lunges
7. 35 lunges
8. 35 lunges
9. 35 lunges
10. Max out: perform as many lunges as you can.

Max reps: _____

If you completed this workout, head to Gorilla Group Workout 6 for your next session. If not, stick with this one until you complete it.

Glasses of water drank today: 1-2-3-4-5-6-7-8-9-10

Hours of sleep last night: 1-2-3-4-5-6-7-8-9-10

Diet: junk food————semi-healthy————healthy

Gorilla Group Workout 6

Welcome to the Gorilla Group Workout 6.

For this workout, you have 10 sets with 90 seconds of rest between each set.

Remember to focus on proper form throughout your sets.

Sets:

1. 37 lunges
2. 37 lunges
3. 37 lunges
4. 37 lunges
5. 37 lunges
6. 37 lunges
7. 37 lunges
8. 37 lunges
9. 37 lunges
10. Max out: perform as many lunges as you can.

Max reps: _____

Since this is the end of a two-week period, it is time to redo your lunge assessment to check your progress if you fully completed this workout.

Rest a day and give the assessment a go to see which Group you will be in next.

Glasses of water drank today: 1-2-3-4-5-6-7-8-9-10

Hours of sleep last night: 1-2-3-4-5-6-7-8-9-10

Diet: junk food—————semi-healthy—————healthy

Viking Group Workouts

Viking Group Workout 1

Welcome to the Viking Group Workout 1.

For this workout, you have 6 sets with 120 seconds of rest between each set.

Remember to focus on proper form throughout your sets.

Sets:

1. 56 lunges
2. 56 lunges
3. 56 lunges
4. 56 lunges
5. 56 lunges
6. Max out: perform as many lunges as you can.

Max reps: _____

If you completed this workout, head to Viking Group Workout 2 for your next session. If not, stick with this one until you complete it.

Glasses of water drank today: 1-2-3-4-5-6-7-8-9-10

Hours of sleep last night: 1-2-3-4-5-6-7-8-9-10

Diet: junk food—————semi-healthy—————healthy

Viking Group Workout 2

Welcome to the Viking Group Workout 2.

For this workout, you have 9 sets with 90 seconds of rest between each set.

Remember to focus on proper form throughout your sets.

Sets:

1. 35 lunges
2. 35 lunges
3. 35 lunges
4. 35 lunges
5. 35 lunges
6. 35 lunges
7. 35 lunges
8. 35 lunges
9. Max out: perform as many lunges as you can.

Max reps: _____

If you completed this workout, head to Viking Group Workout 3 for your next session. If not, stick with this one until you complete it.

Glasses of water drank today: 1-2-3-4-5-6-7-8-9-10

Hours of sleep last night: 1-2-3-4-5-6-7-8-9-10

Diet: junk food—————semi-healthy—————healthy

Viking Group Workout 3

Welcome to the Viking Group Workout 3.

For this workout, you have 9 sets with 90 seconds of rest between each set.

Remember to focus on proper form throughout your sets.

Sets:

1. 37 lunges
2. 37 lunges
3. 37 lunges
4. 37 lunges
5. 37 lunges
6. 37 lunges
7. 37 lunges
8. 37 lunges
9. Max out: perform as many lunges as you can.

Max reps: _____

If you completed this workout, head to Viking Group Workout 4 for your next session. If not, stick with this one until you complete it.

Glasses of water drank today: 1-2-3-4-5-6-7-8-9-10

Hours of sleep last night: 1-2-3-4-5-6-7-8-9-10

Diet: junk food————semi-healthy————healthy

Viking Group Workout 4

Welcome to the Viking Group Workout 4.

For this workout, you have 6 sets with 120 seconds of rest between each set.

Remember to focus on proper form throughout your sets.

Sets:

1. 70 lunges
2. 70 lunges
3. 70 lunges
4. 70 lunges
5. 70 lunges
6. Max out: perform as many lunges as you can.

Max reps: _____

If you completed this workout, head to Viking Group Workout 5 for your next session. If not, stick with this one until you complete it.

Glasses of water drank today: 1-2-3-4-5-6-7-8-9-10

Hours of sleep last night: 1-2-3-4-5-6-7-8-9-10

Diet: junk food—————semi-healthy—————healthy

Viking Group Workout 5

Welcome to the Viking Group Workout 5.

For this workout, you have 10 sets with 90 seconds of rest between each set.

Remember to focus on proper form throughout your sets.

Sets:

1. 41 lunges
2. 41 lunges
3. 41 lunges
4. 41 lunges
5. 41 lunges
6. 41 lunges
7. 41 lunges
8. 41 lunges
9. 41 lunges
10. Max out: perform as many lunges as you can.

Max reps: _____

If you completed this workout, head to Viking Group Workout 6 for your next session. If not, stick with this one until you complete it.

Glasses of water drank today: 1-2-3-4-5-6-7-8-9-10

Hours of sleep last night: 1-2-3-4-5-6-7-8-9-10

Diet: junk food————semi-healthy————healthy

Viking Group Workout 6

Welcome to the Viking Group Workout 6.

For this workout, you have 10 sets with 90 seconds of rest between each set.

Remember to focus on proper form throughout your sets.

Sets:

1. 48 lunges
2. 48 lunges
3. 48 lunges
4. 48 lunges
5. 48 lunges
6. 48 lunges
7. 48 lunges
8. 48 lunges
9. 48 lunges
10. Max out: perform as many lunges as you can.

Max reps: _____

Since this is the end of a two-week period, it is time to redo your lunges assessment to check your progress if you fully completed this workout.

Rest a day and give the assessment a go to see which Group you will be in next.

Glasses of water drank today: 1-2-3-4-5-6-7-8-9-10

Hours of sleep last night: 1-2-3-4-5-6-7-8-9-10

Diet: junk food—————semi-healthy—————healthy

Elite Group Workouts

Elite Group Workout 1

Welcome to the Elite Group Workout 1.

For this workout, you have 6 sets with 120 seconds of rest between each set.

Remember to focus on proper form throughout your sets.

Sets:

1. 66 lunges
2. 66 lunges
3. 66 lunges
4. 66 lunges
5. 66 lunges
6. Max out: perform as many lunges as you can.

Max reps: _____

If you completed this workout, head to Elite Group Workout 2 for your next session. If not, stick with this one until you complete it.

Glasses of water drank today: 1-2-3-4-5-6-7-8-9-10

Hours of sleep last night: 1-2-3-4-5-6-7-8-9-10

ELITE GROUP WORKOUT 1

Diet: junk food—————semi-healthy—————healthy

121

Elite Group Workout 2

Welcome to the Elite Group Workout 2.

For this workout, you have 9 sets with 90 seconds of rest between each set.

Remember to focus on proper form throughout your sets.

Sets:

1. 30 lunges
2. 30 lunges
3. 30 lunges
4. 30 lunges
5. 30 lunges
6. 30 lunges
7. 30 lunges
8. 30 lunges
9. Max out: perform as many lunges as you can.

Max reps: _____

If you completed this workout, head to Elite Group Workout 3 for your next session. If not, stick with this one until you complete it.

Glasses of water drank today: 1-2-3-4-5-6-7-8-9-10

Hours of sleep last night: 1-2-3-4-5-6-7-8-9-10

Diet: junk food—————semi-healthy—————healthy

Elite Group Workout 3

Welcome to the Elite Group Workout 3.

For this workout, you have 9 sets with 90 seconds of rest between each set.

Remember to focus on proper form throughout your sets.

Sets:

1. 43 lunges
2. 43 lunges
3. 43 lunges
4. 43 lunges
5. 43 lunges
6. 43 lunges
7. 43 lunges
8. 43 lunges
9. Max out: perform as many lunges as you can.

Max reps: _____

If you completed this workout, head to Elite Group Workout 4 for your next session. If not, stick with this one until you complete it.

Glasses of water drank today: 1-2-3-4-5-6-7-8-9-10

Hours of sleep last night: 1-2-3-4-5-6-7-8-9-10

Diet: junk food—————semi-healthy—————healthy

Elite Group Workout 4

Welcome to the Elite Group Workout 4.

For this workout, you have 6 sets with 120 seconds of rest between each set.

Remember to focus on proper form throughout your sets.

Sets:

1. 83 lunges
2. 83 lunges
3. 83 lunges
4. 83 lunges
5. 83 lunges
6. Max out: perform as many lunges as you can.

Max reps: _____

If you completed this workout, head to Elite Group Workout 5 for your next session. If not, stick with this one until you complete it.

Glasses of water drank today: 1-2-3-4-5-6-7-8-9-10

Hours of sleep last night: 1-2-3-4-5-6-7-8-9-10

Diet: junk food————semi-healthy————healthy

Elite Group Workout 5

Welcome to the Elite Group Workout 5.

For this workout, you have 10 sets with 90 seconds of rest between each set.

Remember to focus on proper form throughout your sets.

Sets:

1. 48 lunges
2. 48 lunges
3. 48 lunges
4. 48 lunges
5. 48 lunges
6. 48 lunges
7. 48 lunges
8. 48 lunges
9. 48 lunges
10. Max out: perform as many lunges as you can.

Max reps: _____

If you completed this workout, head to Elite Group Workout 6 for your next session. If not, stick with this one until you complete it.

Glasses of water drank today: 1-2-3-4-5-6-7-8-9-10

Hours of sleep last night: 1-2-3-4-5-6-7-8-9-10

Diet: junk food—————semi-healthy—————healthy

Elite Group Workout 6

Welcome to the Elite Group Workout 6.

For this workout, you have 10 sets with 90 seconds of rest between each set.

Remember to focus on proper form throughout your sets.

Sets:

1. 54 lunges
2. 54 lunges
3. 54 lunges
4. 54 lunges
5. 54 lunges
6. 54 lunges
7. 54 lunges
8. 54 lunges
9. 54 lunges
10. Max out: perform as many lunges as you can.

Max reps: _____

Since this is the end of a two-week period, it is time to redo your lunge assessment to check your progress if you fully completed this workout.

Rest a day and give the assessment a go to see which Group you will be in next.

Glasses of water drank today: 1-2-3-4-5-6-7-8-9-10

Hours of sleep last night: 1-2-3-4-5-6-7-8-9-10

Diet: junk food————semi-healthy————healthy

Commando Group Workouts

Commando Group Workout 1

Welcome to the Commando Group Workout 1.

For this workout, you have 6 sets with 120 seconds of rest between each set.

Remember to focus on proper form throughout your sets.

Sets:

1. 70 lunges
2. 70 lunges
3. 70 lunges
4. 70 lunges
5. 70 lunges
6. Max out: perform as many lunges as you can.

Max reps: _____

If you completed this workout, head to Commando Group Workout 2 for your next session. If not, stick with this one until you complete it.

Glasses of water drank today: 1-2-3-4-5-6-7-8-9-10

Hours of sleep last night: 1-2-3-4-5-6-7-8-9-10

Diet: junk food————semi-healthy————healthy

Commando Group Workout 2

Welcome to the Commando Group Workout 2.

For this workout, you have 10 sets with 90 seconds of rest between each set.

Remember to focus on proper form throughout your sets.

Sets:

1. 31 lunges
2. 31 lunges
3. 31 lunges
4. 31 lunges
5. 31 lunges
6. 31 lunges
7. 31 lunges
8. 31 lunges
9. 31 lunges
10. Max out: perform as many lunges as you can.

Max reps: _____

If you completed this workout, head to Commando Group Workout 3 for your next session. If not, stick with this one until you complete it.

Glasses of water drank today: 1-2-3-4-5-6-7-8-9-10

Hours of sleep last night: 1-2-3-4-5-6-7-8-9-10

Diet: junk food—————semi-healthy—————healthy

Commando Group Workout 3

Welcome to the Commando Group Workout 3.

For this workout, you have 10 sets with 90 seconds of rest between each set.

Remember to focus on proper form throughout your sets.

Sets:

1. 46 lunges
2. 46 lunges
3. 46 lunges
4. 46 lunges
5. 46 lunges
6. 46 lunges
7. 46 lunges
8. 46 lunges
9. 46 lunges
10. Max out: perform as many lunges as you can.

Max reps: _____

If you completed this workout, head to Commando Group Workout 4 for your next session. If not, stick with this one until you complete it.

Glasses of water drank today: 1-2-3-4-5-6-7-8-9-10

Hours of sleep last night: 1-2-3-4-5-6-7-8-9-10

Diet: junk food—————semi-healthy—————healthy

Commando Group Workout 4

Welcome to the Commando Group Workout 4.

For this workout, you have 6 sets with 120 seconds of rest between each set.

Remember to focus on proper form throughout your sets.

Sets:

1. 86 lunges
2. 86 lunges
3. 86 lunges
4. 86 lunges
5. 86 lunges
6. Max out: perform as many lunges as you can.

Max reps: _____

If you completed this workout, head to Commando Group Workout 5 for your next session. If not, stick with this one until you complete it.

Glasses of water drank today: 1-2-3-4-5-6-7-8-9-10

Hours of sleep last night: 1-2-3-4-5-6-7-8-9-10

Diet: junk food—————semi-healthy—————healthy

Commando Group Workout 5

Welcome to the Commando Group Workout 5.

For this workout, you have 10 sets with 90 seconds of rest between each set.

Remember to focus on proper form throughout your sets.

Sets:

1. 52 lunges
2. 52 lunges
3. 52 lunges
4. 52 lunges
5. 52 lunges
6. 52 lunges
7. 52 lunges
8. 52 lunges
9. 52 lunges
10. Max out: perform as many lunges as you can.

Max reps: _____

If you completed this workout, head to Commando Group Workout 6 for your next session. If not, stick with this one until you complete it.

Glasses of water drank today: 1-2-3-4-5-6-7-8-9-10

Hours of sleep last night: 1-2-3-4-5-6-7-8-9-10

Diet: junk food—————semi-healthy—————healthy

Commando Group Workout 6

Welcome to the Commando Group Workout 6.

For this workout, you have 10 sets with 90 seconds of rest between each set.

Remember to focus on proper form throughout your sets.

Sets:

1. 58 lunges
2. 58 lunges
3. 58 lunges
4. 58 lunges
5. 58 lunges
6. 58 lunges
7. 58 lunges
8. 58 lunges
9. 58 lunges
10. Max out: perform as many lunges as you can.

Max reps: _____

If you completed this workout, you have earned the right to attempt hitting 200 consecutive lunges. Take a few days off to fully recover and take a shot at

hitting your goal.

You got this.

Glasses of water drank today: 1-2-3-4-5-6-7-8-9-10

Hours of sleep last night: 1-2-3-4-5-6-7-8-9-10

Diet: junk food————semi-healthy————healthy

Veteran Group Workouts

Veteran Group Workout 1

Welcome to the Veteran Group Workout 1.

For this workout, you have 6 sets with 120 seconds of rest between each set.

Remember to focus on proper form throughout your sets.

Sets:

1. 86 lunges
2. 86 lunges
3. 86 lunges
4. 86 lunges
5. 86 lunges
6. Max out: perform as many lunges as you can.

Max reps: _____

If you completed this workout, head to Veteran Group Workout 2 for your next session. If not, stick with this one until you complete it.

Glasses of water drank today: 1-2-3-4-5-6-7-8-9-10

Hours of sleep last night: 1-2-3-4-5-6-7-8-9-10

Diet: junk food—————semi-healthy—————healthy

Veteran Group Workout 2

Welcome to the Veteran Group Workout 2.

For this workout, you have 10 sets with 90 seconds of rest between each set.

Remember to focus on proper form throughout your sets.

Sets:

1. 45 lunges
2. 45 lunges
3. 45 lunges
4. 45 lunges
5. 45 lunges
6. 45 lunges
7. 45 lunges
8. 45 lunges
9. 45 lunges
10. Max out: perform as many lunges as you can.

Max reps: _____

If you completed this workout, head to Veteran Group Workout 3 for your next session. If not, stick with this one until you complete it.

Glasses of water drank today: 1-2-3-4-5-6-7-8-9-10

Hours of sleep last night: 1-2-3-4-5-6-7-8-9-10

Diet: junk food————semi-healthy————healthy

Veteran Group Workout 3

Welcome to the Veteran Group Workout 3.

For this workout, you have 10 sets with 90 seconds of rest between each set.

Remember to focus on proper form throughout your sets.

Sets:

1. 52 lunges
2. 52 lunges
3. 52 lunges
4. 52 lunges
5. 52 lunges
6. 52 lunges
7. 52 lunges
8. 52 lunges
9. 52 lunges
10. Max out: perform as many lunges as you can.

Max reps: _____

If you completed this workout, head to Veteran Group Workout 4 for your next session. If not, stick with this one until you complete it.

Glasses of water drank today: 1-2-3-4-5-6-7-8-9-10

Hours of sleep last night: 1-2-3-4-5-6-7-8-9-10

Diet: junk food—————semi-healthy—————healthy

Veteran Group Workout 4

Welcome to the Veteran Group Workout 4.

For this workout, you have 6 sets with 120 seconds of rest between each set.

Remember to focus on proper form throughout your sets.

Sets:

1. 106 lunges
2. 106 lunges
3. 106 lunges
4. 106 lunges
5. 106 lunges
6. Max out: perform as many lunges as you can.

Max reps: _____

If you completed this workout, head to Veteran Group Workout 5 for your next session. If not, stick with this one until you complete it.

Glasses of water drank today: 1-2-3-4-5-6-7-8-9-10

Hours of sleep last night: 1-2-3-4-5-6-7-8-9-10

Diet: junk food————semi-healthy————healthy

Veteran Group Workout 5

Welcome to the Veteran Group Workout 5.

For this workout, you have 10 sets with 90 seconds of rest between each set.

Remember to focus on proper form throughout your sets.

Sets:

1. 58 lunges
2. 58 lunges
3. 58 lunges
4. 58 lunges
5. 58 lunges
6. 58 lunges
7. 58 lunges
8. 58 lunges
9. 58 lunges
10. Max out: perform as many lunges as you can.

Max reps: _____

If you completed this workout, head to Veteran Group Workout 6 for your next session. If not, stick with this one until you complete it.

Glasses of water drank today: 1-2-3-4-5-6-7-8-9-10

Hours of sleep last night: 1-2-3-4-5-6-7-8-9-10

Diet: junk food————semi-healthy————healthy

Veteran Group Workout 6

Welcome to the Veteran Group Workout 6.

For this workout, you have 10 sets with 90 seconds of rest between each set.

Remember to focus on proper form throughout your sets.

Sets:

1. 66 lunges
2. 66 lunges
3. 66 lunges
4. 66 lunges
5. 66 lunges
6. 66 lunges
7. 66 lunges
8. 66 lunges
9. 66 lunges
10. Max out: perform as many lunges as you can.

Max reps: _____

If you completed this workout, you have earned the right to attempt hitting 200 consecutive lunges. Take a few days off to fully recover and take a shot at

hitting your goal.

You got this.

Glasses of water drank today: 1-2-3-4-5-6-7-8-9-10

Hours of sleep last night: 1-2-3-4-5-6-7-8-9-10

Diet: junk food————semi-healthy————healthy

Nuclear Group Workouts

Nuclear Group Workout 1

Welcome to the Nuclear Group Workout 1.

For this workout, you have 6 sets with 120 seconds of rest between each set.

Remember to focus on proper form throughout your sets.

Sets:

1. 99 lunges
2. 99 lunges
3. 99 lunges
4. 99 lunges
5. 99 lunges
6. Max out: perform as many lunges as you can.

Max reps: _____

If you completed this workout, head to Nuclear Group Workout 2 for your next session. If not, stick with this one until you complete it.

Glasses of water drank today: 1-2-3-4-5-6-7-8-9-10

Hours of sleep last night: 1-2-3-4-5-6-7-8-9-10

Diet: junk food————semi-healthy————healthy

Nuclear Group Workout 2

Welcome to the Nuclear Group Workout 2.

For this workout, you have 10 sets with 90 seconds of rest between each set.

Remember to focus on proper form throughout your sets.

Sets:

1. 52 lunges
2. 52 lunges
3. 52 lunges
4. 52 lunges
5. 52 lunges
6. 52 lunges
7. 52 lunges
8. 52 lunges
9. 52 lunges
10. Max out: perform as many lunges as you can.

Max reps: _____

If you completed this workout, head to Nuclear Group Workout 3 for your next session. If not, stick with this one until you complete it.

Glasses of water drank today: 1-2-3-4-5-6-7-8-9-10

Hours of sleep last night: 1-2-3-4-5-6-7-8-9-10

Diet: junk food—————semi-healthy—————healthy

Nuclear Group Workout 3

Welcome to the Nuclear Group Workout 3.

For this workout, you have 10 sets with 90 seconds of rest between each set.

Remember to focus on proper form throughout your sets.

Sets:

1. 58 lunges
2. 58 lunges
3. 58 lunges
4. 58 lunges
5. 58 lunges
6. 58 lunges
7. 58 lunges
8. 58 lunges
9. 58 lunges
10. Max out: perform as many lunges as you can.

Max reps: _____

If you completed this workout, head to Nuclear Group Workout 4 for your next session. If not, stick with this one until you complete it.

Glasses of water drank today: 1-2-3-4-5-6-7-8-9-10

Hours of sleep last night: 1-2-3-4-5-6-7-8-9-10

Diet: junk food————semi-healthy————healthy

Nuclear Group Workout 4

Welcome to the Nuclear Group Workout 4.

For this workout, you have 6 sets with 120 seconds of rest between each set.

Remember to focus on proper form throughout your sets.

Sets:

1. 109 lunges
2. 109 lunges
3. 109 lunges
4. 109 lunges
5. 109 lunges
6. Max out: perform as many lunges as you can.

Max reps: _____

If you completed this workout, head to Nuclear Group Workout 5 for your next session. If not, stick with this one until you complete it.

Glasses of water drank today: 1-2-3-4-5-6-7-8-9-10

Hours of sleep last night: 1-2-3-4-5-6-7-8-9-10

Diet: junk food————semi-healthy————healthy

Nuclear Group Workout 5

Welcome to the Nuclear Group Workout 5.

For this workout, you have 10 sets with 90 seconds of rest between each set.

Remember to focus on proper form throughout your sets.

Sets:

1. 66 lunges
2. 66 lunges
3. 66 lunges
4. 66 lunges
5. 66 lunges
6. 66 lunges
7. 66 lunges
8. 66 lunges
9. 66 lunges
10. Max out: perform as many lunges as you can.

Max reps: _____

If you completed this workout, head to Nuclear Group Workout 6 for your next session. If not, stick with this one until you complete it.

Glasses of water drank today: 1-2-3-4-5-6-7-8-9-10

Hours of sleep last night: 1-2-3-4-5-6-7-8-9-10

Diet: junk food————semi-healthy————healthy

Nuclear Group Workout 6

Welcome to the Nuclear Group Workout 6.

For this workout, you have 10 sets with 90 seconds of rest between each set.

Remember to focus on proper form throughout your sets.

Sets:

1. 70 lunges
2. 70 lunges
3. 70 lunges
4. 70 lunges
5. 70 lunges
6. 70 lunges
7. 70 lunges
8. 70 lunges
9. 70 lunges
10. Max out: perform as many lunges as you can.

Max reps: _____

If you completed this workout, you have earned the right to attempt hitting 200 consecutive lunges. Take a few days off to fully recover and take a shot at

hitting your goal.

You got this.

Glasses of water drank today: 1-2-3-4-5-6-7-8-9-10

Hours of sleep last night: 1-2-3-4-5-6-7-8-9-10

Diet: junk food—————semi-healthy—————healthy

Attempting 200 Consecutive Lunges

If you are here, that means you have completed either the Commando, Veteran, or Nuclear Group Workouts and have earned the right to attempt 200 consecutive lunges.

This goal is well within your grasp and all you have to do is take it.

As you begin to warm up to crush this, I'd like to ask a favor.

I'm going to be greedy for a minute here and ask you to leave a review for the book.

Reviews are a pain to get but it will only take a minute or two to leave one.

Scan this QR which will take you straight to the book's page on Amazon.

Scroll down and click the 'leave a customer review' button, select your star rating, leave a few words, and that is it!

It is that simple!

Once that is done, get ready to crush this.

Get psyched for what is about to happen.

Give it everything you have got to knock out as many correct lunges without stopping.

Once you are done, come back.

* * *

If you nailed 200 or more, awesome.

That is incredible. Time to knock that off your bucket list.

If you did not quite get it, no worries. Not everyone gets it on the first try.

Use this number as your new assessment number and get back at it!

Cheers.

Conclusion:

I just want to thank you for making your way through this program and the book. You have bettered yourself for it.

I hope you have challenged yourself and I hope you tasted victory by reaching 200 consecutive lunges.

If you are hungry for more challenges, we've got plenty more where this came from.

And if you have enjoyed this book, do take a second to leave a review.

Until next time.

Cheers.

www.ingramcontent.com/pod-product-compliance
Lightning Source LLC
Chambersburg PA
CBHW022054020426
42335CB00012B/681